The Spanish Flu

The Great Pandemic of 1918. The

Worst Deadliest Influenza of All

Time.

Dr. Peter Gordon

CONTENTS

INTRODUCTION

The Spanish flu, which occurred in 1918, affecting everybody globally, was the deadliest in the history of flu. The virus was highly infectious and surged in a few months. It is believed that the Spanish flu was triggered by H1NI, which caused influenza an infection. The duration of the flu was from the beginning of 1918 to mid-1920, which infected over half a billion people, a time the world's third population. The pandemic happened in three consecutive waves. People estimated 17-50 million lost their lives to this deadliest influenza virus in the history of all human epidemics.

In early 1918, the cause and the spread of human flu, commonly known as influenza A virus of Spanish flu and its associations with swine flu and birds to avian, were mysterious. Despite epidemiologic and clinical resemblances to flu pandemics of 1847, 1889, and even past, many questioned if the fatal disease could be influenza. The question resolved the 1930s when similar viruses, known as H1N1 and related to flu, were isolated from pigs and later from a human being. Subsequently, studies that were done for seroepidemiologic were linked to the 1918 pandemic of both viruses. Consequent research shows that the 1918 virus descendants continue in pigs enzootically.

They constantly circulated in human being, undertaking steady antigenic shift and drift, thus causing the 1950s epidemics. The emergent of Asian Flu (H2N2) in 1957 was directly linked with H1N1 virus-related descendants pandemic strain of 1918, which extincted in people circulation, though the lineage related enzootically in pigs. The H1N1 human virus re-emerged abruptly from a freezer in a laboratory. They endure to move and infect people epidemically and endemically.

CHAPTER 1: SPANISH FLU OF 1918

Flu or influenza is a virus-related respiratory disease that invades the breathing system, including lungs, nose, and throat caused by A and B viruses of flu. It occurs across the globe, which significantly causes mortality and morbidity every year. The Human flu A and B illnesses cause recurrent flu epidemics nearly every single winter in the U.S. Influenza A viral infection are the primary influenza infections that cause influenza or flu pandemics, which is the global flu epidemics disease. A pandemic occurs when different and new flu viruses emerge, contagious to human beings, and affect many people in the continents and across the globe.

Influenza A virus infection is categorized into two types based on the number of proteins on the virus's superficial layer. They include neuraminidase and Hemagglutinin. Both Hemagglutinin and neuraminidase have 18 and 11 subtypes, respectively. With more than 198 different potential influenzas A subtype groupings, only 131 subtypes have been noticed in natural surroundings. The common types of flu viruses that are highly infectious and regularly circulate in human being include A(H3N2) and A(H1N1). Influenza A types are further classified in diverse hereditary clades and sub-clades. Influenza B infections are categorized into two lineages, which include B/Victoria and B/Yamagata. Both influenza A and B viruses subtypes are classified into particular groups and sub-groups commonly referred to as clades and sub-clades.

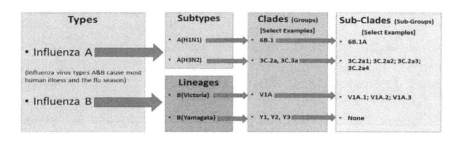

Human seasonal influenza virus. Source: CDC, 2019.

The influenza infection is complicated and continually keeps changing. The influenza virus physical arrangement makes it particularly susceptible to minor surface variations in antigens throughout replication, thus making the virus to equivocate the host's defense mechanism. These make the influenza virus infect and re-infect individuals in the ensuing years due to weak body immunity.

Due to variations of the influenza virus, people's immunity to flu is short-term, making large populations vulnerable to influenza in the ensuing year. The disease is a recurrent infection in moderate weather. Influenza A virus contaminates many different animals, including humans, other mammals, pigs, aquatic birds, and horses, while the influenza B virus infects only humans. Influenza A virus is a zoonotic disease, and from time to time, infections in birds and animals jump and affect humans being.

The 1918 Spanish influenza virus was one of the severe pandemics in recent history. The pandemic influenza virus originated from pigs, while the 1957 and 1968 epidemics were said to have come into being from contact with avian species. The habitant regions of the proximity of pigs, birds, and human being played a crucial role in establishing a conducive environment for antigenic drifts and shifts. It is imperative to have an exceptional reconnaissance in such regions.

The Spanish flu presented different signs and symptoms, including fever, higher in children, cough, chills, runny nose, sore throat, muscle ache, headache, and frequently extreme weakness. The virus is contagious, spread mainly through aerosols(airborne), and overcrowding in enclosed spaces. Most people who get infected with the influenza virus recover fully within 1-2 weeks. Nevertheless, severe virus complications can occur, predominantly in older people, children, and other susceptible groups with low immunity due to underlying diseases. The most common possible fatal complication of the influenza virus is bacterial pneumonia, and the other influenza complication is virus-related pneumonia, which is rare but has more severe effects.

The primary method of preventing influenza is by vaccination. Though, due to the continually varying flu viruses composition, the modification of the influenza vaccine each year is a must to match current viruses. These involve getting detailed circulating strains knowledge of different types of influenza viruses—the WHO created an International surveillance network of influenza in 1948 and became in charge of its administration. The administration system comprises 82 countries that have 110 influenza state centers and four other Cooperating Midpoints for WHO Research and Reference on Influenza situated in London,

UK, Atlanta, USA, London, UK, and Tokyo, Japan with possibilities of establishing new centers.

This network assists in monitoring influenza trends globe and ensuring that the information is shared with all WHO were collaborating. The centers' virus is isolated for research and reference for instant identification of any new strain. Selected collaborating centers are mandated to deal with specimens of animals. Influenza results from the influenza network are analyzed every February and September, and approval for the antigenic composition for the subsequent year's vaccine of influenza is prepared by WHO and handed on to the vaccine manufacturers. The review and recommendations of February and September relate to the composition of the vaccine predictable for the northern hemisphere and Southern hemisphere in winter, respectively.

CHAPTER 2: ORIGINS OF SPANISH FLU

The Spanish flu, which occurred in 1918, affecting everybody globally, was the deadliest in the history of flu. The virus was highly infectious and surged in a few months. It is believed that the Spanish flu was triggered by H1NI, which caused influenza an infection. The duration of the flu was from the beginning of 1918 to mid-1920, which infected over half a billion people, a time the world's third population. The pandemic happened in four consecutive waves. People estimated 17-50 million lost their lives to this deadliest influenza virus in the history of all human epidemics.

In early 1918, the cause and the spread of human flu, commonly known as influenza A virus of Spanish flu and its associations with swine flu and birds to avian, were mysterious. Despite epidemiologic and clinical resemblances to flu pandemics of 1847, 1889, and even past, many questioned if the fatal disease could be influenza. The question resolved the 1930s when similar viruses, known as H1N1 and related to flu, were isolated from pigs and later from a human being. Subsequently, studies that were done for seroepidemiologic were linked to the 1918 pandemic of both viruses. Consequent research shows that the 1918 virus descendants continue in pigs enzootically.

They constantly circulated in human being, undertaking steady antigenic shift and drift, thus causing the 1950s epidemics. The emergent of Asian Flu (H2N2) in 1957 was directly linked with H1N1 virus-related descendants pandemic strain of 1918, which extincted in people circulation, though the lineage related enzootically in pigs. The H1N1 human virus re-emerged abruptly from a freezer in a laboratory. They endure to move and infect people epidemically and endemically.

In early 2006, there were two lineage descendant H1N1 virus of 1918, which persisted naturally, a human endemic/epidemic H1N1 lineage, classic swine flu(enzootic H1N1 lineage), and the human lineage H3N2 virus, which lead to porcine H3N2 family. The H3N2 and H1N1 families have been linked with lesser deaths and illnesses than the 1918 virus. However, the H3N2 lineage has been associated with higher deaths than H1N1.

Earlier and later, 1918, most influenza viruses emerged in Asia and spread across the globe. The influenza virus spread in different waves in Asia, North America, and in Europe. The first wave was described in March 1918 in the United States. There is no epidemiologic and historical data to classify the virus's geographical source with the recent genetic analysis of the 1918 virus genome, which does not place the influenza virus in any environmental context.

The 1918 influenza virus A was not reported supposed to be for all reportable diseases, and diagnostic standards for pneumonia and influenza were ambiguous. This lead to the sharp rise of pneumonia and influenza virus-related death in the United States in 1915 and 1916 as the major of a primary lung disease widespread in December 1915. Death rates curved to some extent in 1917.

The 1918 virus pandemic had a sole characteristic, the concurrent contagion of swine and humans. The 1918 influenza A virus pandemic expressed an antigenically new subcategory, to which almost all humans being and pigs were naïve immunologically in 1918. Newly written and printed phylogenetic and sequence analyses put forward that the encoding of genes neuraminidase and hemagglutinin superficial layer proteins of the

1918 infection resulted from birds like the influenza virus before the start of the epidemic. The precursor diseases had not spread to swine and humans in a few years before. In the latest gene segments, analyses of the virus support this assumption. The human and swine flu sequences regression of gene analysis acquired from 1930 to date place the preliminary transmission of the 1918 precursor infection in humans at nearly 1915–1918. As a result, the precursor was most likely not spreading widely to people until in a while before 1918. nor did the virus appear from any avian species, and its origin remains puzzling.

Millions of people succumbed to the influenza virus than those who died during World War 1, which was previously known as the Great War. The flu virus pandemic was devastating documented in modern Global history. Many people succumbed to influenza in one year than Black Death Bubonic disease of four years from 1347 to 1351.

The genesis of the influenza virus is not well known, though the virus comes from China. It is thought to have originated in China in a sporadic genetic drift and shift of the flu virus. The recombination of the virus superficial layer of a protein created a new virus, which leads to the loss of people herd immunity. Lately, reconstruction of the virus from dead soldier tissue is currently being characterized genetically. The name of the influenza virus, commonly known as Spanish flu, came from Spain after massive deaths and the early illness on 10/19/1918. There was no acknowledgment or response to the Spanish flu epidemics in military camps in March and April of 1918. It was unluckily because no single steps or strategies were applied to prepare for the surge and recrudescence of the infectious influenza virus strain in the winter. Due to lack of virus research, Incorrect application of control methods of the virus used and later criticized because the pandemic could not be overlooked in the time of winter in 1918. The military soldiers in the camps were trained on epidemics in 1918.

The viral sequence data recommend that the 1918 virus was new to people, and it was not produced from the existing or old strains of many or one genetics like those which caused pandemics of 1957 or 1968. It is conflicting because the 1918 virus looks like the bird flu/influenza from toto, a mysterious source because its segments of the genome are noticeably diverse from the genes of avian influenza. The wild birds' collected specimens show that approximately the virus DNA segment structures of 1918 show a slight difference from today's avian viruses. These indicate that there are anti genetic variations of avian viruses over extended time in their host.

Viruses which were found in the forest birds had similar gene sequence of 1918 nucleoprotein and the levels of amino acid, but different levels of nucleotide which depicts current nucleoprotein and 1918 nucleoprotein evolution of strains of the wild birds. The development of genes distance can be compared by ratios of identical or non-identical nucleotide substitutions. An equal replacement signifies a silent alteration of a nucleotide modification in a codon that does not replace amino acid. Commonly, a viral genetic factor exposed to an immunologic drift force displays a more significant percentage of non-identical alterations, whereas a virus on slight pressure accrues identical changes. With little or no assorted pressure is applied to identical changes, they reflect the distance of evolution.

With more identical changes of genes segment of the 1918 influenza virus sequence, it was linked with strains of wild birds though they are not likely to have emerged from the influenza virus of birds, which were similar to the sequenced today. It is noted that the 1918 virus sequences have few proteins different from avian strains, which spend a long time adapting in swine or human as the only intermediate host. The influenza virus reservoir has been acquired from rare gene segments that have not been sampled or identified. The genetic material and gene segments of all 1957 and 1968 and 1918 pandemic viruses depicts that the viruses originated from avian viruses of the Eurasian. This lead to the rise of human viruses strain, which was earlier transmitting infection as the H1N1 strain. Analysis of virus gene sequence alone does not substantiate the 1918 virus pathogenicity. Different experiments have been done to give the animal and in vitro model virulence containing 1918 genetic factors using viral constructs by reverse genetics.

Different theories are explaining the origin of the Spanish flu. There is one which describes how the pandemic flu started in Kansas, the United States, and infected human beings from birds. The first case was reported on March 4, 1918, where Army mess cook Albert Gitchell was the first patient. During that time, the

14

Fort Riley camp of U.S. soldiers prepared for World War 1 in the Western Front. The flu was endemic a month later in America Midwest, where they disembarked in the French ports and embarked on eastern seaboard cities.

The other theory explains the rare 1918 flu pandemic virulence by outlining its first outbreak was in Europe's trenches. The virus later declines due to the lack of a host, which made it surge. The 1918 flu could not surge because it erupted in trenches occupied by soldiers who were not traveling. The virus was not virulence due to a lack of evolutionary pressure because it stayed in the trenches for days, weeks, and months. Later, the virus spread and surged in Spain and in Germany soldiers. With the censorship of flu news by war censorship regimes in many countries and Spain thinking that they were the only country enduring the flu outbreak, they got the "Spanish flu" name. The soldiers who were prisoners of war in Russia returned to Germany and spread the disease in the Soviet Union, which was newly created. Other countries in Africa, Japan, India, and China had the outbreak by May and June in 1918.

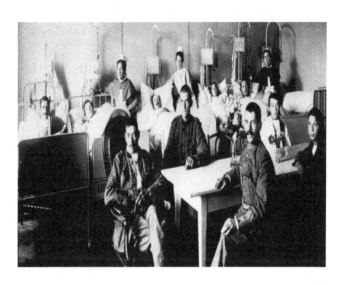

Military hospital with influenza patients in

Switzerland, December 1918

Source: Fox media, 2020

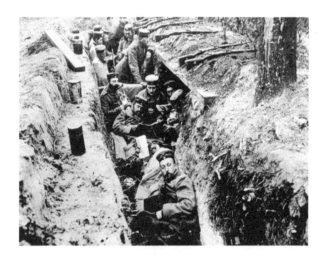

Soldiers in trenches during World War I

Source: Fox media, 2020.

.

CHAPTER 2:1. HOW THE 1918 FLU CURVE WAS FLATTENED

The flattening of the 1918 flu pandemic was done by creating awareness for people to observe physical distancing, which saved many Americans. The first case of the deadly influenza virus in Philadephia was diagnosed on September 17, 1918, fast-spreading. A campaign against coughing, sneezing, and spitting in public was launched by city officials to curb the spread of the deadliest virus. Due to the surge of flu cases, all public gatherings, churches, schools, and theatres were shut down. People who had signs and symptoms of influenza virus were in 1918 quarantined their homes. An increase in population, globalization, and urbanization has made it challenging to contain pandemics. These facilitate fast spread within hours across continents because of similar tools of response. Public Health strategies are applied as the only first line of defense against any pandemic without any vaccine. Different measures used to reduce the spread of any epidemic include country lockdown, closing shops, restaurants, schools, transportation restrictions, physical distancing, and banning all gatherings in public.

Getting people to comply with public health restrictions to limit the spread of pandemics is not easy. Police are used to enforce all laws established by public health, including those found not adhering to the set protocols and guidelines. These helped to cut the infection rate by 30-50%. Some cities, including New York City, closed its borders earlier after the announcement of the Influenza virus. The application of different measures such as allocation of business hours and mandatory quarantine lowered the deaths across the Eastern seaboard.

Everybody feared the virus, and it overwhelmed the hospital's capacity, which they could manage at that time. It killed many people and was the deadliest virus ever experienced up to today. During that time, people were still lagging in the development of vaccines and other drugs for treating various diseases compared to today, where most institutions mandated in drugs and vaccines production have developed their infrastructure.

People were not aware that the virus caused the 1918 influenza. Some people said bacteria caused it until researchers proved that the virus caused it in 1933. Antibiotics were discovered ten years later for treating influenza-related pneumonia.

Medicines capable of managing flu-related pneumonia transmission and the first antiviral medications were developed in 1963—the WHO had not been formed to facilitate tracking and surveillance of severe disease outbreak. Because of war censorship by regimes, most countries across Europe lacked information about the flu outbreak.

The New York state health commissioner ordered the closure of all entertainment places and saloons to stop the spread of influenza, spreading at an alarming rate. In the previous history of epidemics, no drastic actions and strategies were put in place. The deadly influenza virus spread fast across the United States with mysterious characteristics. Similar simultaneous virus emergence was documented in many navies, and army camps with speculation were, their enemies introduced it, and secret service considering it without a doubt. The army said that all people who get access and enter the camps were freezing and which was also under strict surveillance and guarded.

The virus or any other disease can be averted by bursting in the sun and outdoor air. Diseases or germs are contagious to people working in closed stores, workshops, and railroad trains due to bad breath. Hundreds of people attend meeting in a poorly ventilated room except door opening when someone gets in or out. These drastically make the virus spread when one coughs or sneezes in the place. Some people fail to open windows due to the mentality that my neighbor will see what is inside my room, thus making them desist. Prevailing of grip creates employers' production handicap. People working in the workshop should take charge to make sure they are supplied with fresh air. They should wear clothes which are warm to withstand a few drafts. Girls who wear mosquito nets in their waist should substitute during fall weather with something appropriate. Keeping ourselves healthy and physically fit will save fatal illness and other conditions that will help the country run.

People were advised by doctors to avoid other people or crowded places because they were in a hard place and rock with no vaccine for the flu. Other remedies that were also suggested included drinking wine and eating cinnamon, which had no scientific evidence of eliminating the virus. Doctors insisted that people should wear masks to cover their nose and mouth while at public places. Masks could limit the spread of the deadly virus because while talking, one could not spit saliva aerosol, which contains flu virus, which was airborne. By then, Aspirin could be used to cure the infection though it was blamed for causing a pandemic.

Some companies took advantage of the virus and advertised Formamint linking it with symptoms of the Flu in British papers on June 1918, and people noticed it was vitamin tablets. Many companies made fake advertisements promising the cure of the flu, thus creating a lot of money. United States citizens were offered advice of avoiding getting infected. They were highlighted to avoid shaking hands, touching library books, and shaking hands. Theatres and schools were closed, and spitting was made illegal by the Health Department of New York. There was a shortage of doctors as a result of World War I in some areas, and many physicians left contracted the virus and became ill. Most medical colleges, makeshift hospitals, and medical students took the place of doctors who were sick.

Despite the advance in medicine and public health, all measures which were put in place to curb the spread of the deadly influenza virus in 1918 are still instituted today. Different kind of action which were applied then some are used today to manage diseases such as coronavirus. They include quarantine, wearing masks, thorough handwashing for a minimum of 20 seconds, isolation of patients, physical/social distancing, avoiding overcrowding, and locking up of countries, counties, or regions with the surge of the pandemic to limit spreading in the other areas.

These ancient techniques are also applied today, and people now understand that health and sick people have to be separated.

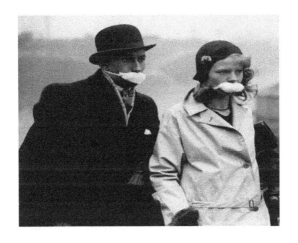

People were poorly wearing masks in 1918

Source: Fox Media, 2019

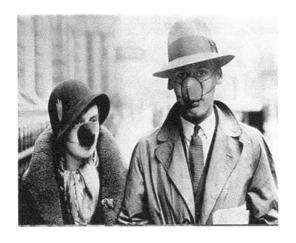

People were correctly wearing masks in 1918.

Source: CDC, 2019

CHAPTER 3: OVERVIEW OF SPANISH FLU

The Spanish flu, commonly known as the strain of the influenza of 1918, caused a deadly global pandemic, killing people indiscriminately and killing people quickly. All those infected by the Spanish flu, including the healthy, old and young, and those with underlying health problems had a 10% death rate.

The virus killed almost 50 million people, a third of the world population in 1918, making it the worst pandemic ever documented. The epidemic gained the Spanish name flu though it was questionable if it originated from Spain. It emerged in 1918 a few months to the end of World War 1. The virus surged and spread quickly because of conflict, which was responsible for the spread of the virus. The soldiers living in dirty and damp and cramped conditions in the Western Front became ill. As a result of malnourishment, their immunity becomes weak. They had highly infectious illnesses, which affected all ranks known as "la grippe" After three days of infection, soldiers felt better though they succumbed because of the virus. As the troops began to return home or leave during the 1918 summer, they spread the virus because they were asymptomatic and later became ill. This lead to the spread of the virus in the soldier's village, cities, and towns in their home countries. Those who have infected both civilians and soldiers did not recover quickly. The virus spread fast in young adults between 20 to 30 who were formerly healthy.

There were some theories on the spread of the virus in 2014, suggesting that it originated in China. There were records undiscovered, which explained how the virus was spread from the Chinese Labour Corps across Canada in 1918. The Chinese laborers were from rural areas who were farmers. They were sealed and transported in train containers in the country for six days and later heading to France. More than 90.000 workers in Western Front were mobilized to excavate furrows, build roads, and damaged tanks repair.

More than 25,000 laborers from Chinese, only 3,000, ended their journey to Canada in medical quarantine in 1918. Due to fallacies stereotypes of race, they blamed Chinese laziness for the illness, and workers' symptoms were not taken seriously by

Canadian doctors. Laborer's who arrived in North France had virus

symptoms, and many were dying in early 1918.

CHAPTER 3.1: WHY WAS INFLUENZA VIRUS NAMED THE SPANISH FLU?

The influenza virus epidemic was first identified in Spain as a result of censorship during the war. The nation of Spain was neutral during the time of war, and strict restrictions on the press were not enforced, which resulted in freely publishing the virus illness information. This lead to people deceptively believing that the influenza virus/flu was specific to Spain hence been named "Spanish flu." During the springtime in 1918, Spain news service sends a message to London, in the U.K., notifying them that they have diagnosed new epidemic disease which had strange characteristics in the capital city, Madrid. No people had died in the time of reporting; however, after two weeks, almost 100,000 contracted the flu.

The deadly virus struck so harder and infected leading politicians and Alfonso XIII, who was the king of Spain. Almost 40% of all living and working in confined areas, including schools, government buildings, and barracks, contracted the virus. The telegraph services were disturbed and reduced track drivers business because many people were sick, and they could not work. Hospitals were overwhelmed and could not keep the demand for people's medical supplies. Spanish influenza was embraced in Britain. British media accused Spanish weather due to the flu surge by communicating that the Spanish windy spring, which was dry, unhealthy season, and unpleasant, facilitated faster spread. It was noted that, due to dusty winds that spread across Spain with microbe-laden, it was stopped by the wet climate of Britain, thus lowered cases of the flu.

CHAPTER 4: ANALYSIS OF THE SPANISH FLU

The influenza virus pandemic of 1918 killed between 20-50 million people globally, including adults and healthy young. The Armed Forces Pathologist from the Institute of Pathology extracted RNA, which was viral in autopsy specimens, and viral genes were sequenced from the victim. Experts in different professions said that the flu pandemic originated from birds to human beings due to the virus's sequence in humans, concerning the 1957 and 1968 influenza virus, viruses involved from the social and avian viral series. The deadliest flu pandemic of 1918 had changes of amino acid, highly pathogenic in the H5N1 bird virus, which succumbed to a lot of people in the past eight years.

The CDC collected data from the Army Forces Institute of Pathology(AFIP) and tested the mice's pathogenicity by recreating the 1918 influenza virus. In comparing the human influenza virus, the deadly 1918 pandemic virus had 40,000 times higher particles of the lung tissue. It had diverse symptoms including, pulmonary edema, inflammation of bronchitis and alveoli, and alveolar of bleeding similar to 1918 human lungs. The team substantiated that the virus changed specific genes by creating viruses that are different from Hemagglutinin being crucial for virulence and polymerase genes. The protein of Hemagglutinin and Hemagglutinin was essential in pathogenesis, occurring in the new virus. The 1918 illness and the H5N1 virus, a novel virus with similar signs and symptoms, have been witnessed, Coronavirus (COVID-19- with over 18 million cases in August 2020 Worldwide and the United States leading with almost 5 million cases and over 158,000 deaths). There is a possibility of other similar flu viruses, which will negatively impact both health and the economy across the globe.

Transfusion of similar viruses can be used to cure people with avian flu pandemic and develop current vaccines and treatment. A recovered patient from the epidemic of bird influenza can donate significant plasma to treat many H5N1 influenza patients. According to a study done by the World Health Organization (WHO), the epidemic of bird influenza can emerge and re-emerge, as reported in 2006 with 141 cases and succumbing to H5N1. The WHO has stated that birds play a critical role in the widespread H5N1 virus, precisely poultry, which is the primary source of Asian infections. High prevalence of the virus in birds surges the probability of bird to people virus transmission. At the point when the virus becomes contagious between human being, leads to epidemic flu. If the virus is infectious, it will move faster, and without antiviral tablets or vaccines, it will surge worldwide.

Many researchers work as a team to identify the heritages and structure of the Spanish flu virus. It took years for them and other virologists to succeed. In mid-1990, Dr. Jeffrey Taubenberger and his team carried out phylogenetic and sequence analysis of 1918 flu genes and recognized that the H1N1, which caused the Spanish flu, originated from birds. Dr. Terrence Tumpey was working to identify virus gene sources in BSL3 improved laboratory situations. It included the use of a suit, double gloves, powered air-purifying respirator (PAPR), and working inside the Class II biosafety cabinet (BSC).

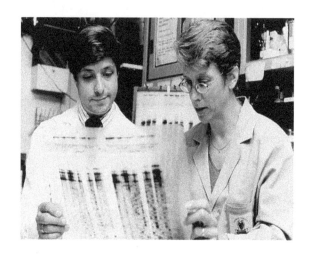

Dr. Jeffery Taubenberger and Dr. Ann Reid reviewing a genetic sequence from the 1918 virus. Source: CDC, 1998

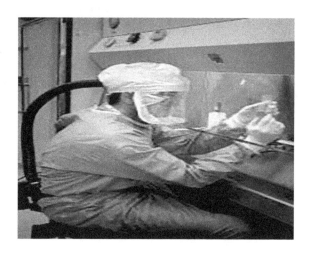

Dr. Terrence Tumpey working in BSL3 enhance laboratory conditions. Source: James Gathany, 2019.

There is a recent development with improved knowledge and capacity to examine viral mutants created by pathogenicity in different experiments. New vaccines have been developed and used to treat mutant pathogens.

CHAPTER 5: CAUSES OF SPANISH FLU

This devastating disease wiped out about 3.3% of the world population in addition to infecting over 30% of humanity. It was caused by a novel pathogen, H1N1, a viral agent with genes derived from birds. The disease spread throughout the world like wildfire between 1918 t0 1919. The causative virus, H1N1, was unique in the sense that it caused high mortality of healthy individuals aged between 15 to 34 years, reducing life expectancy in the USA by over 12 years. Its protein coat made of Hemagglutinin (H.A.) coded by the H.A. gene is essential in the entry and infection of the virus in healthy cells. Antibodies of the immune system also recognize and target the H.A. of the virus. Upon sequencing the virus, it became clear that the ancestors of the virus-infected the human race from 1900 to 1915. By 1918 the virus had gone through several adaptations to become more social and swine-like in its phylogenetic development and diversity. Notably, the virus had been mutating in mammalian hosts before attaining the ability to cause a pandemic. Some alterations in influenza virus genes regularly occur as the virus replicates in a process called antigenic drift, which explains the recurrence of flu seasons annually. Antigenic drift also explains why individuals catch the flu many times in their lifetime. Despite lacking cleavage sites present in modern strains of virulent influenza strains, the Spanish flu virus was highly destructive, a feature associated with many genetic factors. One of the elements is its Neuraminidase (N.A.) gene, which codes for its Neuraminidase coat proteins. It has a significant contribution to the spread of the infection by facilitating its exit from infected cells and attacking healthy cells.

Even if scholars agree that the virus causing the pandemic originated from the bird's family naturally, the precise pathway from its origin until it attained its pandemic nature is mainly elusive. Further, specific genetic factors that can be associated with its extraordinary virulence have not been forthcoming despite several years of intensive research. One school of thought proposes that the pandemic might have begun in Etaples within a British military base in the Northern part of France during the First World War. This key military base housed 100, 000 soldiers in an area of 12km2 characterized by sea marshes occupied by several migratory birds. Nearby multiple farms existed having geese, ducks as well as pigs utilized as the soldiers' food, with horses used for transport. It is believed that the interaction of congested troops, various animals with 24different mutagenic war gases, may have sparked the outbreak of the first epidemic beginning December 1916 to March 1917.

However, other scholars believe that the pandemic may have originated from china—the transportation of Chinese laborers during World War 1 in Canada in sealed trains. Medical records revealed that over 3000 out of the 25000 Chinese laborers on transit in Canada on their way to Europe were later put on quarantine after developing flu-like symptoms. Many Chinese laborers working behind British and French soldiers in the war front are thought to have been the pandemic's source. The significantly low death rates in China served as evidence of the proposal since it indicated higher immunity levels possibly activated by prior contact with the pandemic virus, H1N1. Besides, historical evidence of a respiratory illness reported in the northern part of china in 1917 was found to be significantly similar to Spanish flu. However, since the influenza virus exists in numerous forms that keep mutating from time to time, it later became extremely challenging to trace its origins. Speculations that the virus that caused the pandemic was manufactured in the lab for use as a biological weapon has also made efforts to determine its source, a daunting venture. A consensus is that an enormous reservoir of similar viruses exists in domestic and wild animals with the potential to transform pandemic type pathogens through a natural reassortment process of its genetic material or human influence.

CHAPTER 6: THREE WAVES OF SPANISH FLU

The pandemic, which took the world as a storm spread in a wave-like manner with three main peaks, characterized enormous death rates. The need to establish processes and mechanisms responsible for the multiple waves of pandemics cannot be ignored. Researchers have proposed viral evolution with effects on transmission or escape form immune responses or both environmental variation and behavioral alterations, among other possible causes of the waves. The Spanish flu pandemic occurred in three different waves, with the last one causing mortality even in 1920.

The pandemic's initial wave struck in 1918 spring. Health officials in Kansas USA first reported the illness in a military facility. The military camp was housing the First World War troops. When the American forces entered Europe, shortly afterward, Spain reported individuals with the disease symptoms in the middle of May. Since Spain maintained neutrality during the war, its press reported the spread of the infection without any restriction resulting in the name Spanish flu. During this phase, one of the central regions of the range included Madrid, mainly due to the San Isidro festive activities occurring at the time. Many people got infected during this wave, including King Alfonso XIII. To contain its spread, the government put stringent confinement measures in place, including stopping of postal services, among other services. The wave persisted for sixty days with a mortality rate of about 0.65 per thousand globally except Australia and South America, which remained free from the pandemic.

The next wave of Spanish flu took place during the autumn season of 1918, with much worse effects than the first wave. Several views have been proposed on how it spread. One of the opinions is that the returning home of soldiers from the war in the summertime was behind the spread; others are of the idea that the Portuguese people going back home by train were the cause of the range, while other believe a mutation of the causative virus was to blame. During the second wave, mortality rates soared, summer festivals were stopped, and religious groups were required to stop activities that could make people realize how few they were. In Zamora, the mortality rate was threefold that of the rest of Spain, mainly due to church activities, which increased its spread. The wave more doctors were infected than the initial surge, with the range and severity getting worse globally. Many proposals exist regarding where this phase began with thoughts revolving around f Liberia, Boston city, and Brest's port, among other possible epicenters. Despite being unaffected during the first phase, Australia became one of the most hit countries, reporting over 80000 deaths, mainly due to soldiers returning from the war-front in Europe.

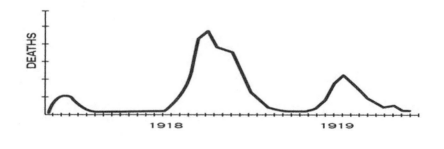

Year

The third wave struck in the early days of the year 1919 and was not as devastating as the second wave because most individuals in the population had gained immunity against the virus. This phase lasted for a more extended period with some countries like Japan reporting cases in 1920. Over eight million individuals had passed away by the time the pandemic ended in Spain. Kids aged 1-3 years old and young adults between 21 and 30 were the most affected individuals. Even though the origin of the virus was never confirmed, three cities were proposed, including Shanxi in China, Etaples in France, and Haskell in the United States of America. The tendency of this virus type to spread in wave-like spikes has made it necessary for healthcare staff to consider pathogens causing similar infections as frequently emergent diseases. In the same century, at least three related pandemics have occurred, including H1N1 in 1918, H2N2 in 1957, and H3N2 of 1968.

CHAPTER 7: EFFECTS ON MAJOR AMERICAN CITIES AND ITS DEVASTATION

Towards the end of summer in 1918, the second phase of the Spanish flu had far-reaching effects on many major American cities. The spike was mainly attributed to returning soldiers from the war Europe. The pandemic initially hit Boston, then New York and Philadelphia before spreading westwards to St. Louis and San Francisco. At the end of the epidemic, about 675000 Americans had died. American cities reported varied levels of the devastation caused by the plague, with cities executing timely and well-organized responses managing to flatten infection and mortality curves. Cities with slow or poorly coordinated responses bore the brunt of the outbreak. On September 28, a Liberty Loan parade in Philadelphia attended by thousands of people resulted in an unprecedented spike of the epidemic. It led to the filling to the capacity of all the 31 health facilities in the state within 72 hours 2600 deaths after one week. Due to the magnitude of the devastation caused by pandemic, massive resources have been allocated to fund research meant to investigate how pandemics arise and practical techniques of mitigating their effects.

An example of a city that responded in a timely and organized manner to flatten the infection curve in St. Louis. Before reporting the pandemic's first case, the city's health commissioner directed health workers to be on high alert and publicized the importance of keeping off from crowded places. When the flu spread from a military camp into the general population, the commissioner did not hesitate to close schools, pool halls, movie theatres, and outlaw public assemblies. These and other measures ensured that the peak death percentage in St. Louis was merely eighth of cases reported in Philadelphia, the U.S. On the other hand, San Francisco enforced the wearing of masks, hoping that it would help flatten the infection curve. The regulation eventually became law with anyone found in public without a cover was charged $5. However, it later became apparent that the gauze masks that were thought to be 99 percent effective in offering protection against the virus were ineffective. Never the less the city recorded relatively low infection rates attributed to the closure of learning institutions, the prohibition of public gatherings as well as the closure of entertainment joints. San Francisco was worst hit in the third wave of the pandemic in January 1919 when the public who mostly believed it was wearing masks that protected them rebelled against social gathering regulations leading to one of the highest mortality rates.

The USA is one of the countries that experienced some of the worst effects of this pandemic. It caused devastating effects so adverse that they are evident even today. Currently, research is still ongoing to unravel the intricacies of the causative pathogen. Burial activities significantly spiked during the fall season, with one family of 12 residing in Pleasant Unity losing eight members in just one week. The deaths caused by the pandemic affected those left behind in psychological, economic, social ways. Children who lost their parents or guardians to the epidemic were left with no option but to fend for themselves.

Moreover, the pandemic seemed to perpetuate disparities in conditions underlying various sections of society, such as health conditions, cultural inequality, war, slavery, crowding, and poverty. The subtle balance between the H1N1 virus and the host dynamics and social factors have been significantly influential in focusing transmission patterns, mechanisms of spreading, and the pandemic's health effects. The epidemic further offered valuable lessons o strategies of handling future pandemics through community, government, and family response measures meant to flatten infection curves, especially of the Covid 19. Containing epidemics depends on the timely, well organized, and collective efforts by all those involved. Any attempts to safeguard personal, business or religious interest would only result in the spiking of infections and subsequent devastating effects on the family, health systems, government services as well as economic prospects of the whole society.

CHAPTER 8: CONSEQUENCES OF THE SPANISH FLU

1. Deaths

It is estimated that Spanish flu murdered 2.7% of people globally. High mortality rate happened between the 20-40 years, as shown in graph 1—the lower the age, the higher the mortality rate. The epidemic took place in three sessions; it initially took place in the summer of 1918, succeeding during the end of 1918, and the final during the initial months of 1919. The second period from October to December 1918 recorded a high mortality rate compared to the first Spanish flu session from July to September 1918. The third session of the Spanish flu was moderately small. The statistics that took place in some cities of England, the United States, and Norway (Vaughan 1921; Great Britain Ministry of Health 1920; Hanssen 1923; Collins 1931; Britten 1932) show a clear picture of how Spanish flue affected individuals based on age-sex. The research shows that influenza impacted negatively on individuals during the summer session.

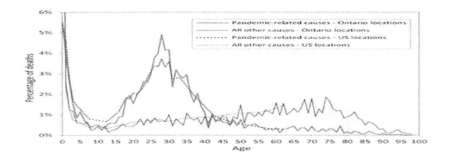

Source: Commonwealth Bureau of Census and Statistics,1920.

High mortality rates were seen in countries such as India, which had a large number of population. Research shows that a high mortality rate was observed in weighted countries than those countries with less weighted.

2. Mental and health disorders

Individuals who survived the epidemic were observed to have disorders such as depressions, dizziness, low blood pressure, sleeping, heart problems, ear illness, hepatitis, deafness, blindness, baldness, and lung tuberculosis. Furthermore, people who survived Spanish flue developed sleeping sickness disorder (encephalitis lethargica). The sleeping sickness was common among youths (10-30 years), and the case is more prone in men than in women. Besides, approximately one million individuals of the world

47

population were infected by Spain flue, and it was reported that half of the people died of the sleeping sickness in the bout 1919-1928. In the case of Norway, 268 cases and 52 deaths were announced. However, the figure of Norway (1.0) tends to be low per 1000 as compared to Sweden (3.0) and Denmark (5.9). It was reported that Spanish influenza survivors developed coronary heart disease (CHD) in their later life. After 1920, men recorded a high number of individuals who had infected with coronary heart disease as compared to women. Correspondingly, Spanish influenza increased cases of alcohol consumption and suicides, and this resulted from increased psychological health disorders. The major causes of suicides were social isolation that resulted from the closure of schools, churches, theatres, and so on. Furthermore, the loss of relatives and couples from Spanish influenza took part in many suicides.

3. Shortage and rationing

During the Spanish influenza epidemic, some foods were rationed due to scarcity and inflation. Youths were significantly affected due to malnutrition and weight loss in the year 1918. The session of rationing resulted in the loss of lives among teenagers, which directly influenced future generations.

4. Mass emigration and selection

The migration of men 1920s built a selection mechanism as women were left behind. For instance, Norway, males, and females born in 1865-85 were decreased by 30 and 20 percent because of emigration.

5. Deterioration of the economy.

In October 1918, there was a decrease in 40- 70 percent in sales departmental stores and merchants in the United States. Similarly, there was a decrease in Gross Domestic Product per capita by about 6 percent in classic countries in a session of 19187-1921. Spanish flu reduced the manufacturing productivity of the United States by 18%. Many industry sectors declined due to the scarcity of labor caused by high mortality rates that left fewer individuals to provide the workforce.

6. Loss of Employment

In Australia, 25- 40 percent of retailers collapsed due to the Spanish flu epidemic. These caused unemployment as most businesses relocated to unaffected areas. Besides, some companies reduced employees due to reduced orders.

7.   Social isolation

Typical countries had quarantine response to prevent the high spread of influenza. Isolation of individuals made their family members feel like they have been isolated.

CHAPTER 9: TREATMENT OF SPANISH FLU

During the 1918 epidemic, physicians did not have any idea about Spanish flue treatment. Medical physicians took the flue to be caused by *Bacillus influ*enza. They separated the types of bacteria under a microscope, which they called microscopic agents. In the 18th century, vaccines for small agents had been discovered. The discovery process took another step in 1931. Richard Shope conducted a study on a pig that had swine flu by applying the same procedures used earlier on discovering causes of yellow fever.

In 1936, Richard discovered that people who associate with pig gardens had a closeness with swine disease. Moreover, complicated innovations went to Vanderbilt University. Scientists were able to identify two common flu viruses, namely A and B. After identifying viruses, researchers started to discover new vaccines in the 1930s to treat the flu. The use of vaccine influenza started working on soldiers in the United States in 1944 and went on to civilians in 1945.

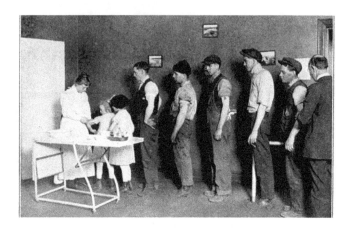

After the research on the vaccine, results showed that one virus's immunity counteracted the other's immunity.

Epidemiological studies indicated the importance of wearing facemasks, which prevented Spanish flu from spreading from host to unaffected one. Influenza A can be treated on its own by having some rest. In some cases, the medical physician may instruct individuals to use Zanamivir, oseltamivir, and peramivir. Fortunately, prescriptions prevent Virus A from spreading within cells. However, they cause vomiting and nausea. One should visit a doctor if the situation persists. There was an invented medicine known as baloxavir marboxil (Xofluza) from a Japanese pharmaceutical company. The dose was accredited in the United States in 1918 under the Food and Drug Administration (FDA). The vaccination tends to be the best method for preventing influenza. The spread of disease may also be prevented through handwashing, avoiding overcrowding, the use of flexed elbow when coughing or sneezing, avoiding unnecessary traveling after being infected by fever, and 24 hours after recovery. Virus A is the most dangerous infection that may cause death if not well treated.

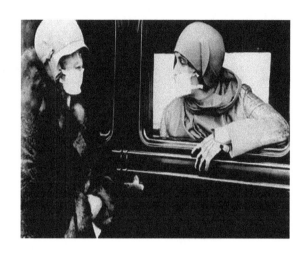

San Francisco residents wearing masks, which Protected the surge

of the virus. Source: Fox media, 2020.

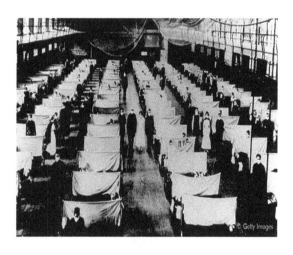

Philadelphia Hospital with Spanish Flu Patients. Source: Fox

media, 2020.

CHAPTER 10: HISTORICAL LESSONS FROM THE SPANISH FLU 1918

The Spanish flu 1918 was the deadliest pandemic that ever happened in the twentieth century. The historical point of view caused over fifty million deaths, with over five hundred million infected with the virus. The disease is known to be caused by a virus known as the H1N1 influenza infection. The essay will highlight the historical lessons that are evident from the Spanish flu pandemic.

One of the first cases to be reported was in the state of Kansas. The individual infected with the disease was a cook known as Albert Gitchel. The common symptoms that he had been coughing, headache, and fever. Three weeks after one of the first cases, it was noted that over one, those U.S. soldiers were hospitalized because of the virus infection. In Europe, the disease spread like fire, with most of the European countries being affected. These were a significant setback of the military operations that were carried out during the first world war. The viral disease infected more than half of both the French and British military troops. North Africa and India reported their first cases in May. However, China and Australia reported their first cases in June and July, respectively. It had flu-like symptoms, but they were mild. The disease caused an increase in the mortality rates during the 1918 to 1920 period.

It had two waves, the first and the second waves. However, the second wave was the deadliest in comparison to the first wave. The first wave of the virus infection, the symptoms were similar to those of influenza though mild. However, the second wave was a mutated strain of the virus, which was first established in the South England port. The second wave lasted close to two months as both the American continents were infected with the inclusion of the west and south African countries. Thus by the end of September, the disease had spread in all European countries. It had begun to spread in Asia with major countries like Russia, India, and China affected in October. As early as November the state of New York, the epidemic was over. However, it persisted in European countries.

The main reason why it persisted in European nations was due to food shortages and fuel shortages. Most cases were reported during the second wave. The second wave is when there was the highest death report as a result of the disease infection. The mutated strained virus's symptoms were very severe, and they included pneumonia, high temperatures of forty degrees, nasal bleeding, coma, and blood-streaked urine. The most affected groups were the military tugs influencing their war strategies. The disease did not spare those of high social class in the society as the king of Spain was afflicted. Towards the end of December, the world was free from the Spanish flu.

The third wave began and originated from Australia. Australia lifted its quarantine measures in January 1919. More than twelve thousand Australian s were infected with the viral disease. By the end of January, the third wave had reached Europe, North America, and South America continents. The third wave was the finals; fewer people were affected compared to the previous waves. By May 1919, the third wave was declared to have finished. Japan experienced its third wave later in the year 1919 and lasted until 1920.

There was clarity about the etiologic of the infection as health authority had issued a worldwide communication. The Pfeiffer Bacillus was not always easy to isolate in the healthcare laboratories. Hemophilia influenza was first discovered by a biologist who found it in the nasal mucus of the patient towards the end of the 19th century.

The Haemophilus bacterium was the causal agent of influenza. Two scientists advanced further research of then pathogen that is responsible for the flu infection. The pathogen that was discovered after the advanced hypothesis was a virus. However, the virus pathological effects advanced to the secondary, which were lethal. This advancement to the secondary level would weaken the body's immunity and cause co-infections such as obesity, measles, and malaria. The Spanish flu infected all age groups; however, the age groups that were mist vulnerable were the Elderly and the children, due to the lack of cross-reactive antibodies that could fight the virus. Due to this issue, the disease spread faster as people were easily infected. The flu pandemic caused between the year 1918 and 1920 was discovered to be a virus in 1930. Three years later, the human influenza virus was successfully isolated.

Several public measures were undertaken to contain the disease from spreading. As there was no cure for the illness, improvised treatment s were implemented to wid those who were infected. Some of the events contributing to the spread included the return of military troops, women engagement in Extra domestic activities, and the refugee migration. The preventive measures were introduced by health authorities to mitigate as well as contain the disease. The first measures were introduced in August 1918. The measures included regular notification and surveillance of communities. European nations further increased restrictions to contain the virus. They closed down public meeting facilities and suspension of public meeting functions. Cleaning and disinfection of the streets, public places, and public facilities helped reduce the virus's surge. The health authorities believed that the open spaces and facilities were considered the cornerstone of the spread of the disease. European health authorities further introduced other measures such as limitation of the number of passengers in public transport and banning of crowd gathering outside shopping centers and other centers. However, these measures did not prove to be effective.

Health organizations provided clean water and soap for the underprivileged in society. The public health department invested in services such as removal of human waste, food products regulations, and toilet regulation. Spitting on the public was prohibited. At the same time, the therapeutic virtues and importance of water were advertised in leaflets and newspapers. European nations such as Italy set up collection centers for corpses as rituals practiced during the death were abolished to contain the spread of the Spanish flu. Quarantine measures were still in effect to contain the disease as no antiviral and vaccine were available to cure the disease.

Spain was not involved in the first world war as it was neutral. The press in Spain had the freedom to report what was happening in their nation concerning the pandemic's effects. It was perceived that the virus originated from Spain and thus earned the name Spanish flu. The Spanish newspapers front page would print the names of those who died if the flu in the front page. However, other European nations avoided reporting news that was related to the pandemic. The reason why other countries avoided saying the communication concerning the epidemic was to avoid alarming the citizens. Towards the end of August 1918, an Italian minister denied the alarming reports of the pandemic to avoid creating alarm to the public. However, the following months to come, both the national and international newspapers avoided reporting the pandemic matter to protect the public from the alarming information. Later on, local hygiene authorities did not disclose the number of individuals who were infected, stringent the health authorities had assured that the disease would not last for not more than two months. However, the condition persisted, and thus the police were under pressure wince the disease was still spreading, and no antiviral or vaccine had been discovered. And thus, the health authorities were under pressure to substantiate their initial claims.

The 1918 influenza had a unique characteristic: it expressed an antigen subtype that the human body immunity was naive to fight against the genes originated from the avian-like influenza virus. They include neuraminidase and Hemagglutinin. Were determined as precursors of the disease as they were discovered in the year 1915 to 1918 before the pandemic. However, for the influenza virus infection to occur, there needs to be a binding of the sacs acid receptors found on the surface of the cell and the H.A protein. The hemagglutinin receptors that infect the birds differ in terms of configuration with those that affect the human immune system.

The Spanish flu was a global health catastrophe as it was associated with a high mortality rate. The disease is said to kill over fifty million people are and the world. The youthful age group was highly affected in terms of the killing as they were categorized between the age of 15 years to 34 years. Due to the pandemic, life expectancy was lowered. The degree of mortality and morbidity never repeated in the event the disease reoccured in 1957 and 1968. This revealed that the health authorities were able to contain the disease and learn from the historical measures. However, this raised a question of why the disease was a major pandemic during the 1918 to 1920 period. Various reasons evolved, and they include the state of living during the time and the war. The virus at the time had a unique characteristic that was responsible for the high spread among humans. The virus was never isolated during 1918 because of the lack of modern medical technology known as tissue culture techniques. However, by using the tissue culture techniques, eight viral genes were discovered using tissue samples obtained from humans who were infected during the period. Under close research after the virus was genetically sequenced, there were no determinants of high virulence.

There are three known antigenically pandemic influenza virus of different subtypes which includes, H1N1 1918, H3N2 1968, and H2N2 1957, which have caused different pandemics. The viruses lacked immunity at the time of the infection. The major one is that if 1918 that caused a global health catastrophe. The 1918 virus is subject to interest since its origin was based on the homology sequence. The homology is the combination of two H.A. of human origin and swine origin. The amino acids that were retrieved from the polymerase proteins of the H1N1 virus looked similar to the avian influenza sequence. The only difference incurred after a phylogenetic analysis is the ten polymerase proteins alterations of amino acid.

63

Scientists perceived that the cause of the epidemic was due to the poor quality of the consumed food. The food consumption was law as the first. World war had created food shortages. However, countries that were not involved in the war, such as Spain, ruled out malnutrition and rationed food products. The other perspective was that the disease was triggered by a war bacteria designed by the Austro-German enemy. Emergency measures were being publicized on how to contain the disease. Some of these measures include the ban on public gathering and shutdown public places such as the cinemas. The news agency had to keep advertising this as they sensitize the public. Since they were to avoid publicizing the turmoil that the pandemic had caused to the nation. The death bells were prohibited from protecting the public from the devastating information concerning the pandemic. The disease caused major upheavals in the social structure in that it took the young population were as made the children to be orphaned.

The 1918 H1N1 virus was reconstructed by DNAs corresponded viral RNA aided of reverse genetics. However, through the reverse genetics influenza virus was rescued from the plasmid DNA. The experiment was carried in mice, and it revealed how the virus was lethal to the specimen. High virulence occurred because of the combination of the polymerase, Hemagglutinin (H.A), and Neuraminidase (N.A) genes.

The H.A. gene is a glycoprotein of the influenza virus its responsible for fusion of the host's endosomal membrane with the viral envelope. The H.A. is also the receptor-binding protein and requires the host protein enzyme protease to be triggered, which splits the H.A. genes into two subunits. The NA gene also encodes a glycoprotein, which is viral that contradicts the H.A. However, the N.A. mediates the viral release by cleaving the viral receptors.

Five hundred million were infected by the disease, whereas the disease had caused fifty million deaths. The most affected were the military troops in the first world war as it produced over a hundred thousand graves of military forces. This was the highest mortality rate of Americans in Europe as a result of the disease. It is also revealed that the virus-infected over one million American troops. Several factors and activities were shown to have caused the severe spread, and they include overcrowding, flies, dust, and length of military service. Overcrowded camps, the chances of the flu being spread were high, and thus the Military troops were profoundly affected by the disease. Bacterial pneumonia, the secondary effect level of Spanish influenza 1918, was the real cause of high mortality among those infected with the virus. It's challenging to clarify the mortality rate resulting from the disease as statistical research centers fail to submit complete information concerning the issue. In Italy, complete data concerning the military were infected was revealed. Through the report, the researchers were able to project accurate data of those who died because of the pandemic. The military medical team was repeatedly subjected to the virus. However, during the second wave, most military health workers were infected and caused a high mortality rate.

Preparation of future pandemics, influenza brought a toll on the healthcare system in terms of measures to be adopted to contain the disease. Flu still is a health threat as it plans to adapt to immunologically susceptible humans that might occur as antigen drift if antigen shift.

Preparation is very crucial in response to a future influenza outbreak. The pandemic had taught the health authorities they must integrate measures during the early phase to contain and eliminate the disease. In case there is no vaccine, then medical supplies for personal protection, social distancing measures, antibiotics, and antivirals should be administered in place.

CHAPTER 11: CONCLUSION

To conclude, the Spanish flu 1918 was the worst health problem that ever occurred since no antiviral was discovered and the vaccine. The disease caused the highest mortality rate in history. The biological analysis of the military personnel who were infected and died remains credible information that research scientists would use to discover new vaccines and antivirals. The data also may be used in creating preventive measures. The information is trustworthy as it will aid in giving insights on how to deal with future pandemics in case they arise. As for the military troops, the Spanish Influenza affected the fighting strength and morale in the war. The data also will aid the medical experts in terms of the appropriate time that one should be administered with the antibiotics. However, the pandemic improved public health and health care organization s around the world. The healthcare authorities invested in many strategies, such as sanitation, surveillance, and health education, to improve public knowledge on the transmission of influenza globally. However, the plans are still being implemented to prevent the spread of the disease. It has played a significant role in history on how health organizations around the world should prepare for if health pandemic occurs in the future.

Dedicated to all of the victims of pandemics, current and past.

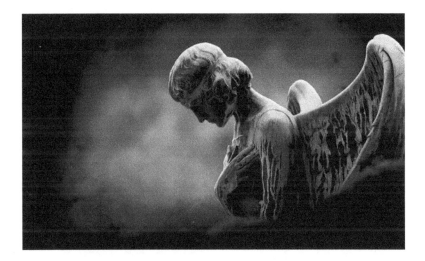